RENAL FUNCTION COOKBOOK

THE ULTIMATE DIET COOKBOOK FOR KIDNEY DISEASE

BETHANY LAKYNN

Table of Contents

CHAPTER ONE

Diet for renal function

A renal or kidney diet must be followed by those with impaired kidney function in order to reduce the amount of waste in their blood. Food and liquids we eat and drink contribute to the buildup of waste in our bloodstreams. Renal dysfunction results in an inability to effectively filter and eliminate waste. The electrolyte balance of a patient can be adversely affected by waste remaining in the blood. A kidney diet may also help to maintain kidney function and slow the progression of renal failure.

Low in sodium, phosphates, and protein is a renal diet. In addition to limiting fluid intake and emphasizing high-quality protein, a renal diet places an emphasis on these other factors. Potassium and calcium restrictions are also necessary for some patients. Because every person's body is unique, working with a renal dietitian to develop a diet specific to each patient is essential.

If I have kidney disease, what kind of diet should I follow?

Controlling sodium, potassium, and phosphorus may be necessary for people with kidney disease. Please talk to your doctor or the dietitian at your dialysis center about your unique dietary requirements. Here are some renal diet guidelines to follow.

Salt contains sodium, which is a mineral (sodium chloride). It's used extensively in the kitchen.

Salt is one of the most common seasonings in the kitchen. Adapting to a lower salt intake will take some time. Reducing salt and sodium intake is critical to managing your kidney disease, however.

To get you started, consider the following ideas.

1.

Don't add salt to your food while cooking.

2.

Never season your food with salt.

3.

Learn how to read the nutrition information on food packages. Don't eat anything with more than 300 milligrams of sodium in each serving (or 600mg for a complete frozen dinner). Keep an eye out for ingredients with salt listed as the fourth or fifth item on the list.

4.

Do not consume pork products like ham, bacon and sausages, hot dogs, lunch meats, chicken tenders, or nuggets. Restrict your intake of soups with potassium chloride to one cup at a time, rather than the entire can.

5.

The label should read "no salt added" if you're looking for canned vegetables.

6.

Garlic, onion, and seasoned salts should not be used. Use regular table salt only.

7.

Look for low-sodium or no-sodium options for your favorite foods, like peanut butter or box mixes.

8.

Don't buy meat that has been pre-flavored or pre-seasoned, whether it is refrigerated or frozen, that has been packaged in a solution. A wide variety of options are available, including boneless chicken and bone-in chicken pieces as well as turkey breast and whole turkey.

Sodium is a mineral that helps muscles function. It's common for potassium to build up in your blood when your kidneys aren't functioning properly. This can lead to changes in your heartbeat and even a heart attack as a result of this.

Fruits and vegetables, milk, and meats are the main sources of potassium in the diet. Some fruits and vegetables should be avoided, while others should be consumed in moderation.

Foods high in potassium should be avoided.

CHAPTER TWO

- Cantaloupe and honeydew melons. (Watermelon is fine.)"

- Bananas.

In addition, there are oranges and orange juice.

- Avocado.

- Juice from a ripe tree.

Ingredients: • Tomatoes • Tomato Sauce

Dried beans of all kinds.

• Squash in the fall and winter.

Spinach, kale, collards, and Swiss chard are all examples of cooked greens.

• Brussels sprouts and broccoli.

Nuts, including nut butters.

In addition, you should steer clear of the following:

• Granola and bran cereals.

Substitutes for salt such as "lite" salt

• Molasses.

Fruits in a can

Potassium levels in canned fruits are typically lower than those in fresh ones. Before eating the fruit, be sure to drain off any excess juice.

The sweet potato and the potato

The proper handling of potatoes and sweet potatoes necessitates the consumption of only small amounts of them. Soak them for several hours in a large amount of water after peeling and cutting them into small slices or cubes.

The soaking water should be drained before cooking, and a large amount of water should be used. Prepare your food by removing this water.

If I'm on a renal diet, what should I be aware of regarding phosphorus in my diet?

One of the minerals that can build up in the blood when

kidneys aren't working properly is phosphorus. Your skin and blood vessels may become filled with calcium when this happens. Bone disease can then become an issue, increasing your risk of breaking a bone.

Recommendations for reducing phosphorus intake

Limit your consumption of milk to one cup per day, as dairy foods are the primary source of phosphorus in the diet. If you choose to substitute liquid milk with yogurt or cheese, limit yourself to one container or 1.5 ounces of cheese per day.

Phosphorus is also found in a number of vegetables. Limit your intake to no more than one cup per week:

• Beans in their natural state.

• Greens.

• Broccoli.

• Mushrooms.

This includes brussel sprouts.

- Bran.

- Wheat-based foods.

- Oatmeal.

- Granola.

The phosphorus in white or Italian bread and low-salt crackers made with white flour is lower than the phosphorus in whole-grain bread and crackers..

Soft drinks contain phosphorus, so stick to the clear variety.

There is also phosphorus in beer. Avoid them all.

There are 17 foods you should avoid or limit if your kidneys are in poor health.

They are bean-shaped organs that do a lot of important things.

They're in charge of everything from blood filtering to waste removal via urine, hormone production, mineral balance, and fluid balance maintenance.

Kidney disease can be caused by a wide range of factors. Most common are diabetes and high blood pressure that are not being properly controlled by the patient.

Hepatitis C and HIV are also known to contribute to kidney disease.

Fluid can build up in the body and waste can accumulate in the blood if the kidneys are damaged and unable to function properly.

If you want to improve kidney function and prevent further kidney damage, you may want to limit or eliminate certain foods from your diet.

Kidney disease and poor eating habits

As kidney disease progresses, so do the dietary restrictions.

As an example, people in the early stages of chronic kidney

disease will have different dietary restrictions than those in the final stages of renal failure.

End-stage renal disease patients who are on dialysis are subject to a variety of dietary restrictions, as well. Dialysis is a medical procedure that removes excess water and filters waste.

Most people with advanced kidney disease must adhere to a kidney-friendly diet in order to prevent blood levels of certain chemicals or nutrients from becoming too high.

CHAPTER THREE

Patients with chronic kidney disease are unable to remove excess sodium, potassium, or phosphorus from the blood because their kidneys are unable to do so. Consequently, they are at greater risk of having elevated levels of these minerals in their bloodstreams

When it comes to a kidney-friendly diet, sodium, potassium, and phosphorus intake are all restricted to less than 2,300 mg per day.

The most recent Kidney Disease Outcomes Quality Initiative (KDOQI) guidelines from the National Kidney Foundation do not specify a potassium or phosphorus intake limit for patients.

When it comes to potassium and phosphorus, kidney disease patients should consult with a doctor or dietitian to determine their personal limits, which are usually based on laboratory results.

The waste products of protein metabolism may also be difficult to filter if the kidneys are damaged. If you're on dialysis, you should limit the amount of protein you eat unless you have chronic kidney disease in stages 3–5.

End-stage renal disease dialysis patients have an increased protein requirement'

On a renal diet, there are 17 foods you should probably avoid.

1. Soda that is dark in color

Soda contains phosphorus-containing additives, especially dark-colored sodas, in addition to the sugar and calories they contain.

Adding phosphorus to processed foods and drinks can improve flavor, extend shelf life, and prevent discoloration, all of which are important considerations for consumers.

Phosphorus supplements are better absorbed by your body than natural, animal- or plant-based phosphorus.

Unlike naturally occurring phosphorus, which is protein-bound, additive phosphorus is not. Rather, it is found in the form of salt, which is easily absorbed by the digestive system.

The ingredient list of a product usually contains additive phosphorus. Food manufacturers, on the other hand, are not required to disclose the exact amount of phosphorus in their products.

For most dark-colored sodas, the amount of phosphorus in a

200-mL serving is estimated to be between 50 and 100 mg, depending on the brand.

A 12-ounce can of Coca-Cola has 33.5 milligrams of phosphorus in it, according to the USDA food database.

As a result, on a renal diet, sodas should be avoided, particularly those that are dark.

Phosphorus, which is highly absorbed by the human body in its additive form, can be found in dark-colored sodas.

2. Avocados

Academias are often praised for their numerous health benefits, including their heart-healthy fats, fiber, and antioxidants.

Avocados are generally good for you, but if you have kidney disease, you should stay away from them.

Potassium is abundant in avocados, which is why they're so good for you. There are 690 mg of potassium in a medium-sized avocado.

People with kidney disease can still eat avocados, but they can limit their potassium intake by consuming only one-fourth of an avocado per meal.

On a renal diet, avocados, including guacamole, should be restricted or avoided if potassium intake is a concern. As long as you keep in mind your overall diet and health goals as the most important consideration, you should be fine.

If your doctor or nutritionist has advised you to reduce your potassium intake, you may want to avoid avocados on a renal diet.

3. Preserved food

Soups, vegetables, and beans in cans are popular due to their low cost and ease of use.

However, salt is commonly used as a preservative to extend the shelf life of canned foods.

People with kidney disease should avoid or limit their intake of canned goods because of the high sodium content.

It's usually best to choose sodium-free or "no salt added" varieties.

Canning foods such as beans and tuna and draining and rinsing them can reduce their sodium content by 33–80 percent.

4. Bread made with whole wheat flour

For people with kidney disease, picking the right bread can be a challenge.

CHAPTER FOUR

Whole wheat bread is frequently recommended over refined white flour bread for healthy individuals.

Because of the higher fiber content in whole wheat bread, it may be a healthier option. White bread, on the other hand, is usually recommended for people with kidney disease.

Because of its high phosphorus and potassium content, it is a good source of these minerals. The higher the phosphorus and potassium content, the more bran and whole grains the bread contains.

Whole wheat bread, for example, has 57 mg of phosphorus and 69 mg of potassium in a 30-gram serving. Comparatively, only 28 mg of phosphorus and potassium are found in white bread.

You don't have to give up whole wheat bread completely to reduce your potassium and phosphorus intake by eating one slice instead of two.

Salt is found in almost all bread and bread products, regardless of whether they're made from white or whole-wheat flour (15Trusted Source).

It's a good idea to compare the nutrition labels of different breads, choose a lower sodium option, and keep an eye on your portion sizes.

Due to its lower phosphorus and potassium content, white bread is typically recommended over whole wheat bread on a renal diet. Because sodium is present in all breads, it's best to compare the sodium content of various brands before making a purchase.

5. a type of rice called brown rice

In terms of potassium and phosphorus content, brown rice is similar to whole wheat bread in that it is an entire grain.

Phosphorus (150 mg/cup) and potassium (154 mg/cup) are found in cooked brown rice, but only 69 mg/cup in cooked white rice.

Brown rice can be included in a renal diet, but only if the serving size is kept in check and balanced with other foods to avoid a daily potassium and phosphorus intake that is too high.

In addition to brown rice, couscous and pearled barley are nutritious, low-phosphorus grains that can be substituted for couscous.

This type of rice is likely to be restricted on a renal diet due to its high phosphorus and potassium content. It's possible to make this dish with any of a number of different grains instead of brown rice.

6. Bananas

For their high potassium content, bananas are a popular choice.

When it comes to sodium content, a medium banana contains 422 mg of potassium.

If a banana is a regular part of your diet and you've been told to watch your potassium intake, it may be difficult to stick to that regimen.

Because of the high potassium content of many other tropical fruits, this can be a problem.

The potassium content of pineapples, on the other hand, is much lower compared to that of other tropical fruits, making them a healthier alternative.

It is possible that bananas, which are high in potassium, should be restricted on a renal diet. Unlike other tropical fruits, pineapple has a low potassium content, making it a good choice for people with kidney disease.

7. Dairy

Vitamin and nutrient content abounds in dairy products.

In addition, they are a good source of protein, phosphorus, and potassium.

When it comes to whole milk, for example, it contains 349 mg potassium (222 mg phosphorus).

In people with kidney disease, excessive consumption of dairy and other phosphorus-rich foods can have a negative impact on bone health.

Although it may come as a shock to some, milk and other dairy products are frequently recommended for building strong bones and maintaining healthy muscles.

A buildup of phosphorus in your blood can cause calcium to be pulled from your bones when your kidneys are damaged by too much phosphorus consumption. You may be at greater risk of bone breakage or fracture as a result of this.

Additionally, dairy foods contain a lot of protein. Whole milk has about 8 grams of protein per cup (240 mL).

To avoid the buildup of protein waste in the blood, it may be necessary to limit dairy consumption.

As a result of their low potassium, phosphorus and protein content, unenriched rice milk and almond milk can be used in place of milk while on the renal diet.

Sodium, phosphorus, potassium, and protein are all found in dairy products and should be restricted on a renal diet. Phosphorus in milk can weaken bones in people with kidney disease, despite the high calcium content of milk.

8. Indulge in some citrus fruits and juice.

Despite the fact that vitamin C is the most well-known benefit of oranges and orange juice, they also contain a significant amount of potassium.

Potassium content per 184-gram orange is 333 milligrams. Additionally, 1 cup (240 mL) of orange juice contains 473 mg of potassium.

Oranges and orange juice, which are high in potassium, should be avoided or consumed in moderation by those on a renal diet.

CHAPTER FIVE

Because they contain less potassium than oranges, they make excellent substitutes for the fruit and its juice. This includes apples, pears, and cranberries, as well as their juices.

Potassium-rich oranges and orange juice should be avoided by those on a renal diet. Instead, consume the juices of grapes, apples, cranberries, or any other of these fruits.

9. Meats that have been processed

Preservative-laden processed meats have long been linked to chronic illness and are generally considered unhealthy.

Salted, dried, cured, or canned meats are all examples of processed meats.

An example of this is hot dogs with bacon, pepperoni or jerky as well as sausages and bacon jerky.

Salt is commonly found in high concentrations in processed meats, primarily for the purposes of enhancing and preserving flavor.

As a result, if processed meats are a regular part of your diet, it may be difficult to stay under 2,300 mg of sodium per day.

As a bonus, processed meats are an excellent source of protein.

If you've been told to keep an eye on your protein intake, it's also a good idea to avoid processed meats.

A renal diet should limit consumption of processed meats, which are high in sodium and protein.

10. Relish, olives, and pickles all fall into this category.

There are many examples of cured or pickled foods such as canned pickles, canned olives, and canned relish.

Curing or pickling typically involves the addition of a significant amount of salt.

More than 300 mg of sodium can be found in just one pickle spear. Sweet pickle relish, on the other hand, contains 244 mg of sodium in 2 tablespoons.

In addition to being salty, cured and fermented olives tend to be less bitter. There are 195 milligrams of sodium in just five green pickled olives, which is a large portion of the daily intake in a small serving.

Preservatives such as sodium are widely available in grocery stores as reduced sodium versions of traditional pickles, olives, and relish.

Although reduced-sodium options can still be high in sodium, you'll still want to keep an eye on your portion sizes.

On a renal diet, limit the intake of sodium-rich foods like pickles, processed olives, and relish.

11. Apricots

Apricots are a good source of vitamin C, vitamin A, and dietary fiber, among other nutrients.

In addition, they are a good source of potassium. The potassium content of one cup of fresh apricots is 427 mg.

Furthermore, dried apricots have a higher potassium content than fresh apricots.

More than 1,500 mg of potassium can be found in one cup of dried apricots.

Just one cup of dried apricots provides 75% of the 2,000-mg potassium limit.

On a renal diet, apricots, especially dried apricots, should be avoided.

On a renal diet, stay away from apricots because of their high potassium content. They provide more than 400 mg in 1 cup of raw material and more than 1,500 mg in 1 cup of dried material.

12. The sweet potato and the potato

There is a lot of potassium in sweet potatoes and regular potatoes.

Potassium content per medium baked potato (156 grams) is 610 mg, while the potassium content per medium baked sweet potato (114 grams) is 541 mg.

It's possible to reduce the amount of potassium in some foods by soaking or leaching them, including potatoes and sweet potatoes.

Potassium content can be reduced by half by boiling potatoes for at least 10 minutes after cutting them into small, thin pieces.

At least four hours before cooking, potatoes that have been soaked in water are proven to be even lower in potassium than those that haven't been soaked.

The double-cooking method, or potassium leaching, is the name given to this process.

It's important to remember that, despite the fact that double cooking potatoes reduces their potassium content, this method does not eliminate their potassium content.

Portion control is the best way to keep potassium levels in check when eating potatoes that have been double-cooked.

Potassium-rich foods include potatoes and sweet potatoes. Potassium content in potatoes can be reduced by half when they are boiled or twice when they are double cooked.

13. Tomatoes

Another fruit with a high potassium content that may not be suitable for a renal diet is the tomato.

Cooking with them is common, as they can be eaten raw or stewed.

Potassium levels in a single cup of tomato sauce can reach as high as 900 milligrams (35).

Tomatoes are a common ingredient in many dishes, which is unfortunate for those on a renal diet.

CHAPTER SIX

For those who prefer a lower potassium alternative, the choice is up to them. But a roasted red pepper sauce can be just as delicious and provide less potassium per serving than tomato sauce.

On a renal diet, tomatoes and other high-potassium fruits and vegetables should probably be avoided.

14. Packaged, ready-to-eat, and microwaveable meals

Sodium levels in the diet can be largely attributed to processed foods.

They are the most heavily processed of the foods on this list and thus contain the most sodium.

Frozen pizza, microwaveable meals, and instant noodles are just a few examples.

If you eat a lot of highly processed foods, it may be difficult to keep your sodium intake below 2,300 mg per day.

Processed foods are high in sodium and often devoid of essential nutrients.

Consuming pre-packaged, ready-to-eat, and instant meals is a bad idea because they are highly processed and lack essential nutrients like vitamins and minerals. On a renal diet, it's best to avoid these foods.

15. Beet greens, spinach, and Swiss chard all make an appearance.

Leafy greens like Swiss chard, spinach, and beet greens are

high in potassium and other nutrients and minerals.

The amount of potassium in a cup of raw spinach ranges from 140 to 290 milligrams.

The potassium content of cooked leafy vegetables remains the same, despite their reduced serving size.

Half a cup of raw spinach, for example, cooks down to about a tablespoon of spinach. As a result, consuming half a cup of cooked spinach has a higher potassium content than consuming half a cup of raw spinach.

To avoid overconsumption of potassium, eat raw Swiss chard, spinach, and beet greens rather than cooked greens.

However, keep in mind that these foods are also high in oxalates, so limit your consumption. Those who are sensitive to oxalates are more likely to develop kidney stones.

Renal tissue can be further damaged by kidney stones,

resulting in a reduction in kidney function.

A serving of cooked greens, such as Swiss chard, spinach, or beet greens is a great way to get your daily potassium intake. When cooked, the potassium content remains the same, despite the smaller serving sizes.

16. Pistachios, dates, and raisins

Most people are familiar with dried fruits like dates, raisins, and prunes, but there are many others.

All of a fruit's nutrients, including potassium, are concentrated when it is dried.

While the potassium content of prunes is nearly five times greater than the potassium content of raw plums, this is not the only example.

In addition, 4 dates contain 668 milligrams of potassium per serving.

It's best to avoid these common dried fruits, which are high in potassium, if you're on a renal diet and want to make sure your potassium levels stay healthy.

Dehydration concentrates nutrients in fruits. Dried fruit, such as dates, prunes, and raisins, have a high potassium content and should be avoided when following a renal diet.

17. Crackers, pretzels, and chips

Snack foods like pretzels and chips tend to be deficient in nutrients, and they're also a significant source of salt.

Furthermore, because of the ease with which these foods can be eaten in excess of the recommended serving size, people often end up consuming even more salt than they intended.

In addition, potato chips are high in potassium because they are made from potatoes.

The high salt content of snacks like pretzels, chips, and crackers makes them ideal for snacking in large quantities. Potassium is a nutrient that is found in large quantities in potato chips.

The nitty-gritty

The reduction of potassium, phosphorus, and sodium intake can help manage kidney disease if you have it.

Foods high in sodium, potassium, and phosphorus should be limited or avoided, as should those high in calcium and magnesium.

Depending on the severity of your kidney damage, your dietary restrictions and nutrient intake recommendations will change.

It's understandable that a renal diet would be intimidating and constricting at times. A healthcare professional and renal dietitian can help you design a renal diet that is tailored to your specific needs, however..

THE END